C000050899

Deformity: an essay. By William Hay, Esq. The fourth edition.

William Hay

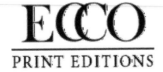

ECCO
PRINT EDITIONS

Deformity: an essay. By William Hay, Esq. The fourth edition.
Hay, William
ESTCID: T129140
Reproduction from British Library

Dublin : printed by George Faulkner, 1754.
42,[2]p. ; 8°

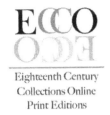

Eighteenth Century
Collections Online
Print Editions

Gale ECCO Print Editions

Relive history with *Eighteenth Century Collections Online*, now available in print for the independent historian and collector. This series includes the most significant English-language and foreign-language works printed in Great Britain during the eighteenth century, and is organized in seven different subject areas including literature and language; medicine, science, and technology; and religion and philosophy. The collection also includes thousands of important works from the Americas.

The eighteenth century has been called "The Age of Enlightenment." It was a period of rapid advance in print culture and publishing, in world exploration, and in the rapid growth of science and technology – all of which had a profound impact on the political and cultural landscape. At the end of the century the American Revolution, French Revolution and Industrial Revolution, perhaps three of the most significant events in modern history, set in motion developments that eventually dominated world political, economic, and social life.

In a groundbreaking effort, Gale initiated a revolution of its own: digitization of epic proportions to preserve these invaluable works in the largest online archive of its kind. Contributions from major world libraries constitute over 175,000 original printed works. Scanned images of the actual pages, rather than transcriptions, recreate the works *as they first appeared.*

Now for the first time, these high-quality digital scans of original works are available via print-on-demand, making them readily accessible to libraries, students, independent scholars, and readers of all ages.

For our initial release we have created seven robust collections to form one the world's most comprehensive catalogs of 18th century works.

Initial Gale ECCO Print Editions collections include:

History and Geography
Rich in titles on English life and social history, this collection spans the world as it was known to eighteenth-century historians and explorers. Titles include a wealth of travel accounts and diaries, histories of nations from throughout the world, and maps and charts of a world that was still being discovered. Students of the War of American Independence will find fascinating accounts from the British side of conflict.

Social Science

Delve into what it was like to live during the eighteenth century by reading the first-hand accounts of everyday people, including city dwellers and farmers, businessmen and bankers, artisans and merchants, artists and their patrons, politicians and their constituents. Original texts make the American, French, and Industrial revolutions vividly contemporary.

Medicine, Science and Technology

Medical theory and practice of the 1700s developed rapidly, as is evidenced by the extensive collection, which includes descriptions of diseases, their conditions, and treatments. Books on science and technology, agriculture, military technology, natural philosophy, even cookbooks, are all contained here.

Literature and Language

Western literary study flows out of eighteenth-century works by Alexander Pope, Daniel Defoe, Henry Fielding, Frances Burney, Denis Diderot, Johann Gottfried Herder, Johann Wolfgang von Goethe, and others. Experience the birth of the modern novel, or compare the development of language using dictionaries and grammar discourses.

Religion and Philosophy

The Age of Enlightenment profoundly enriched religious and philosophical understanding and continues to influence present-day thinking. Works collected here include masterpieces by David Hume, Immanuel Kant, and Jean-Jacques Rousseau, as well as religious sermons and moral debates on the issues of the day, such as the slave trade. The Age of Reason saw conflict between Protestantism and Catholicism transformed into one between faith and logic -- a debate that continues in the twenty-first century.

Law and Reference

This collection reveals the history of English common law and Empire law in a vastly changing world of British expansion. Dominating the legal field is the *Commentaries of the Law of England* by Sir William Blackstone, which first appeared in 1765. Reference works such as almanacs and catalogues continue to educate us by revealing the day-to-day workings of society.

Fine Arts

The eighteenth-century fascination with Greek and Roman antiquity followed the systematic excavation of the ruins at Pompeii and Herculaneum in southern Italy; and after 1750 a neoclassical style dominated all artistic fields. The titles here trace developments in mostly English-language works on painting, sculpture, architecture, music, theater, and other disciplines. Instructional works on musical instruments, catalogs of art objects, comic operas, and more are also included.

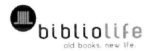

The BiblioLife Network

This project was made possible in part by the BiblioLife Network (BLN), a project aimed at addressing some of the huge challenges facing book preservationists around the world. The BLN includes libraries, library networks, archives, subject matter experts, online communities and library service providers. We believe every book ever published should be available as a high-quality print reproduction; printed on-demand anywhere in the world. This insures the ongoing accessibility of the content and helps generate sustainable revenue for the libraries and organizations that work to preserve these important materials.

The following book is in the "public domain" and represents an authentic reproduction of the text as printed by the original publisher. While we have attempted to accurately maintain the integrity of the original work, there are sometimes problems with the original work or the micro-film from which the books were digitized. This can result in minor errors in reproduction. Possible imperfections include missing and blurred pages, poor pictures, markings and other reproduction issues beyond our control. Because this work is culturally important, we have made it available as part of our commitment to protecting, preserving, and promoting the world's literature.

GUIDE TO FOLD-OUTS MAPS and OVERSIZED IMAGES

The book you are reading was digitized from microfilm captured over the past thirty to forty years. Years after the creation of the original microfilm, the book was converted to digital files and made available in an online database.

In an online database, page images do not need to conform to the size restrictions found in a printed book. When converting these images back into a printed bound book, the page sizes are standardized in ways that maintain the detail of the original. For large images, such as fold-out maps, the original page image is split into two or more pages

Guidelines used to determine how to split the page image follows:

• Some images are split vertically; large images require vertical and horizontal splits.
• For horizontal splits, the content is split left to right.
• For vertical splits, the content is split from top to bottom.
• For both vertical and horizontal splits, the image is processed from top left to bottom right.

DEFORMITY:

AN

ESSAY.

By WILLIAM HAY, Efq;

——— *Te confule , dic tibi quis fis ·*
——— *E cælo defcendit* γνωθι σιαυλον
Juv. Sat. ii.

The Fourth Edition.

DUBLIN:

Printed by GEORGE FAULKNER in *Effex-Street.*
MDCCLIV.

1505

ADVERTISEMENT.

TO promote the Sale of this Piece, the Publisher was for dedicating it to some reigning Toast: but it was thought more for his Interest to send it into the World with the Motto inscribed on the Golden Apple adjudged to *Venus* : for then a thousand Goddesses might seize it as their own.

�֎֎֎֎֎֎֎֎֎֎֎֎֎֎֎֎֎֎֎֎֎֎֎֎֎֎

DEDICATION.

DETUR PULCHRIORI.

TO THE

GREATEST BEAUTY.

✦✦✦✦✦✦✦✦✦✦✦✦✦✦✦✦✦✦✦✦✦✦✦✦

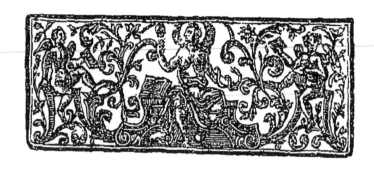

DEFORMITY;

AN

ESSAY, &c.

IT is offensive for a Man to speak much of himself and few can do it with so good a Grace
as *Montaigne* I wish I could, or that I could
be half so * entertaining or instructive My
Subject however will be my Apology· and I am
sure it will draw no Envy upon me. Bodily Deformity is visible to every Eye, but the Effects of it
are known to very few, intimately known to none
but those who feel them, and they generally are
not inclined to reveal them. As therefore I am fur-
nished with the necessary Materials, I will treat this
uncommon Subject at large and to view it in a philosophical Light is a speculation, which may be useful to Persons so oddly (I will not say unhappily) distinguished, and perhaps not unentertaining to others

A 3   I do

---

* The Marquis of *Hallifax* in a Let er to *Charles Cotton*,
Esq, who translated *Montaigne*'s Essays, says, it is the Book in
the World, with which he is best entertained, and that *Montaigne*
did not write for Praise; but to give the World a true Picture of
himself and of Mankind

I do not pretend to be so ingenious as *Montaigne*; but it is in my Power to be as ingenuous. I may with the same * *Naiveté* remove the Veil from my mental as well as personal Imperfections; and expose them naked to the World. And when I have thus anatomized my self, I hope my Heart will be found sound and untainted, and my Intentions honest and sincere

† *Longinus* says, that *Cecilus* wrote of the Sublime in a low Way on the contrary, Mr § *Pope* calls *Longinus* 'The great Sublime he draws' Let it be my Ambition to imitate *Longinus* in Style and Sentiment and, like *Cecilius*, to make these appear a Contrast to my Subject. to write of Deformity with Beauty, and by a finished Piece to atone for an ill-turned Person.

If any Reader imagines, that ‖ a Print of me in the Frontispiece of this Work would give him a clearer Idea of the Subject, I have no Objection, provided he will be at the Expence of ingraving But for want of it, let him know, that I am scarce five Feet high that my Back was bent in my Mother's Womb and that in Person I resemble *Æsop*, the Prince of *Orange*, Marshal *Luxemburg*, Lord Treasurer *Salisbury*, *Scarron*, and Mr *Pope*. not to mention *Thersites* and *Richard* the Third; whom I do not claim as Members of our Society: ** the first being a Child of the Poet's Fancy, the

last

---

* *Vertu Naïve* an Expression of *Montaigne*, and which Fontenelle put into his Mouth in his Dialogue with *Socrates*
† In the Beginning of his Treatise on the Sublime
§ In his Essay on Criticism
‖ It was a disobliging Stroke to a Lady, but it was said of Mademoiselle *de Gournai* that to vindicate her honour from Reflection, she need only prefix her Picture to her Book General Dictionary, under the Word (Gournai)
** *Tam mala Thersiten prohibebat forma latere,*
   Quam pulchrâ Nireus conspiciendus erat
                                    OV Ep. ex Ponto 13 | 4.

laſt miſrepreſented by Hiſtorians, who thought they muſt draw a Devil in a bad Shape. But I will not (on this Occaſion) accept of *Richard*'s Statue from the Hand of any Hiſtorian, or even of *Shakeſpear* himſelf, but only from that of his own * Biographer, who tells (and he ought to know) that *Richard* was a handſome Man.

As I have the greateſt Reaſon to thank God, that I was born in this Iſland, and enjoy the Bleſſings of his Majeſty's Reign, let me not be unthankful, that I was not born in *Sparta* / where I had no ſooner ſeen the Light, but I ſhould have been deprived of it, and have been thrown as a uſeleſs thing † into a Cavern by Mount *Taygetus* / Inhuman *Lycurgus* / thus to deſtroy your own Species ! Surrounded by the Innocents whom you have murdered, may I not haunt you among the Shades below for this Barbarity ? That it was ill Policy, the glorious Liſt of Names, which I have produced, is a Proof your own *Ageſilaus* confutes your Maxim and I hope to confute it too by my own Behaviour Is the Carcaſs the better Part of the Man ? And is it to be valued by Weight, like that of Cattle in a Market ?

Inſtead of this *Lacedemonian* Severity, thoſe, who had the Care of my Infancy, fell into another Extreme ; and, out of Tenderneſs, tried every Art to correct the Errors of Nature, but in vain. for (as I think it is Mr *Dryden* ſays)

' God did not make his Works for Man to mend.'

When they could not do that, they endeavoured

A 4 to

---

* *George Buck*, Eſq, who in his Hiſtory of *Richard* the Third endeavours to repreſent him as a Prince of much better Shapes (both of Body and Mind) than he had been generally eſteemed And Biſhop *Nicolſon* calls *Buck* a more candid Compoſer of Annals than Sir *Thomas More* See his *Hiſtorical Library*.
† See *Plutarch* in the Life of *Lycurgus*.

to conceal them and taught me to be afhamed of my Perfon, inftead of arming me with true Fortitude to defpife any Ridicule or Contempt of it This has caufed me much uneafinefs in my younger Days and it required many Years to conquer this Weaknefs, of which I hope now there are but little Remains left This ill Management gave me too an infuperable Bafhfulnefs and although I have paffed the Courfe of my whole Life among the better Part of Mankind, I have always felt a Reluctance to produce a bad Figure. which may be fome Obftruction to a Man's Advancement in the World. but an Advantage in reftraining his Fondnefs for it.

Unmerited Reflections on a Man's Perfon are hard of Digeftion Men of Underftanding have felt them Even Mr *Pope* was not invulnerable in this Part. For when the Dunces were foiled by his Writing, they printed a Caricatura of his Figure and it is evident that this ftung him more than a better Anfwer for * he ranks it among the moft atrocious Injuries I never in my Life received the leaft Affront on this Head from any Gentleman I ever converfed with, or from any one who had the leaft Pretenfion to that Name for I fhould be a Churl indeed, if I efteemed as fuch any little innocent Pleafantry of a Friend, which is rather an Inftance of fincere Kindnefs and Affection and I fhould be unfit to fit at a Table with him, fhould I refent his Congratulations on my emerging from an Eclipfe of a Surloin of Roaft-beef, or of a Bowl of Punch, that ftood between us But the Scene changes extremely when I get into a Mob, where Infolence grows in Proportion, as the Man finks in Condition and where I can fcarce pafs without hearing

---

* In his Epiftle to Dr *Arbuthnot* are thefe Lines,

The Morals blacken'd, when the Writings 'fcape,
The libelled Perfon, and the *pictur'd Shape,* &c

hearing some Affront. But I am how unmoved with that Scurrility, which used to affect me when I was young Their Title of Lord I never much valued, and now I entirely despise and yet they will force it upon me as an Honour, which they have a Right to bestow, and which I have none to refuse This Abuse is grown into such a Habit with the Rabble, that an *Irish* Chairman often uses it, when he asks me to take a Chair, and sometimes a Beggar when he demands an Alms

This Difference of Behaviour towards me hath given me the strongest Idea of the Force of Education, and taught me to set a right value upon it. It is certainly the Stamp of a Man's Character · it distinguishes the base from the valuable Metal, and is the Barrier between the Mob and the civilized Part of Mankind. This Usage hath also been a great Advantage to me for it hath made me (like * *Horace*) fly from the Vulgar to the Company and Conversation of my Superiors, where I am sure to be easy I have ever enjoyed it, and though I want polite Qualities to recommend me, I cannot say, I was ever ill received by them Moreover, these Abuses from my Inferiors often furnish me with generous Reflections I sometimes recollect the Expression of *Brutus* in *Shakespear*, ' Your ' *Words* pass by me as the idle Wind, which I re- ' gard not ·' at other Times a † Saying (I think) of *Socrates*, ' Shall I be angry if an Ass kick at me ? ' It is his Nature so to do ' But personal Reflections of this kind are almost unknown among Persons of high Rank It must therefore be only a *French* Romance, that gave rise to the Report, that

our

---

* Odi profanum vulgus, & arceo. Ode 1 .l. 3

† I might add another Bon Mot of *Socrates*, when asked, how he could bear the Noise and Ill manners of *Xantippe*, he replied, They that live in a trading Street are not disturbed at the Passage of Carts See the Spectator, N°. 479.

our great and glorious Deliverer once called *Luxemburg* crooked-back Fellow: who replied, that he *could* not know that he was so, for he had never seen his Back

When by some uncommon Accident I have been drawn into a Country Fair, Cock-pit, Bear-garden, or the like riotous Assemblies, after I have got from them, I have felt the Pleasure of one escaped from the Danger of a Wreck for all the Time I am present, I consider myself as liable to Affront, without a Power of shewing any Resentment; which would expose me to ten-fold Ridicule. Nor am I formed for a Masquerade, where such a Figure would soon be discovered, nor escape Abuse from the lower Class, whom the Mask introduces to their Betters; and where all indulge a greater Liberty of Behaviour.

I always had an Aversion in my Childhood to Dancing-masters · and studied all Evasions to avoid their Lessons, when they were forced upon me: for I was ever conscious to myself, what an untoward Subject they had to work on I carried this a little too far, and have sometimes wished I had sacrificed a little more to the Graces The Neglect of this has left behind it an Awkwardness in some Part of my outward Gesture and behaviour and I am sensible, that I might by Care and Habit have corrected some Things now grown inveterate, and that from a natural Dislike to Trifles I neglected some Forms too much

Bodily Deformity is very rare · and therefore a Person so distinguished must naturally think, that he has had ill Luck in a Lottery, where there are above a thousand Prizes to one Blank Among 558 Gentlemen in the House of Commons I am the only one that is so. Thanks to my worthy Constituents, who never objected to my Person; and I hope never to give them Cause to object to my Behaviour

haviour. They are not like a venal Borough, of which there goes a Story, that, though they never took Exceptions to any Man's Character, who came up to their Price, yet they once rejected the best Bidder, because he was a Negroe.

I never was, nor ever will be a Member of the * Ugly Club and I would advise those Gentlemen to meet no more. For though they may be a very ingenious and facetious Society, yet it draws the Eyes of the World too much upon them, and theirs too much from the World For who would chuse to be always looking at bad Pictures, when there is so great a Collection to be met with of good ones, especially among the Fair Sex who, if they will not admit them to be Intimates, will permit them to be distant Admirers. When deformed Persons appear together, it doubles the Ridicule, because of the Similitude, as it does, when they are seen with very large Persons, because of the Contrast Let them therefore call *Minerva* to their Aid in both Cases.

There are many Great and Tall Men, with whom I shall always esteem it an Honour to converse: and though their Eyes are placed in a much higher Parallel, they take Care never to overlook me and are always concerned, if by Chance they happen to strike my Hat with their Elbow When standing or walking we indeed find some Difficulty in the Conversation, for they are obliged to stoop down, as in search of a Pin, while I am looking up, as if taking the Height of a Star with a Quadrant and I own I sometimes use a little Policy, that the Contrast may not be too remarkable.

General *O—w* is Brother in Blood and in Worth to one of the greatest and best Men of the Age · and a brave Spirit is lodged in a large Person. The Man, who stood intrepid by his Majesty's Side in the

the glorious Day of *Dettingen*, and afterwards by that of his Royal Highness in the more unfortunate one of *Fontenay*, is now placed at the Head of a Troop of Horse Grenadiers, to guard that Prince; whom he hath so long and faithfully served. I have the Honour to be well known to him and I once accidentally accompanied him to see the Horses of his Troop I never was more humbled, than when I walked with him among his tall Men; made still taller by their Caps I seemed to myself a Worm and no Man and could not but inwardly grieve that when I had the same Inclination to the Service of my Country and Prince, I wanted their Strength to perform it ——As a Member of the House of Commons, I sometimes use the Precaution to place myself at some Distance from the General, though I am commonly of the same Side of the House.

Lord *D—l—r* is another brave Officer at the Head of one of his Majesty's Troops of Guards and one of the tallest of his Subjects an ancient Peer· an able Senator and (what is much to the Honour of any Peer) a useful Magistrate in the Country I am always proud of meeting his Lordship at the Quarter Sessions but I always take care to have the Chairman at least between us on the Bench, that it may not be too visible to the Country, what a prodigious Disparity there is in every respect between us

But I will now divide my Text, in order to discuss it more thoroughly and will consider the natural Consequences of Bodily Deformity, first, how it affects the outward Circumstances, and lastly, what turn it gives to the Mind

It is certain, that the Human Frame, being warped and disproportioned, is lessened in Strength and Activity, and rendered less fit for its Functions *Scarron* had invented an Engine to take off his Hat, and I wish I could invent one to buckle my Shoe, or to take up a Thing from the Ground, which I

can

can ſcarce do without kneeling, for I can bend my Body no farther than it is bent by Nature For this Reaſon, when Ladies drop a Fan or Glove, I am not the firſt to take them up and often reſtrain my Inclination to perform thoſe little Services, rather than expoſe my Spider-like Shape And I hope it will not be conſtrued as Pride, if I do not always riſe from my Seat when I ought for if it is low, I find ſome Trouble in it, and my Center of Gravity is ſo ill placed, that I am often like to fall back. Things, hanging within the Reach of others, are out of mine ; and what they can execute with Eaſe, I want Strength to perform I am in Danger of being trampled on, or ſtifled, in a Crowd, where my Back is a convenient Lodgment for the Elbow of any tall Perſon that is near. I can ſee nothing · and my whole Employment is to guard my Perſon. I have forborne to attend his Majeſty in the Houſe of Peers, ſince I was like to be ſqueezed to death there againſt the Wall. I would willingly come thither when his Majeſty commands, but he is too gracious to expect Impoſſibilities. Beſides, when I get in, I can never have the Pleaſure of ſeeing on the Throne one of the beſt Princes, who ever ſate on it Theſe and many others are the Inconveniencies continually attending a Figure like mine They may appear grievous to Perſons not uſed to them ; but they grow eaſier by Habit and though they may a little diſturb, they are not ſufficient to deſtroy the Happineſs of Life, of which, at an Average, I have enjoyed as great a Share as moſt Men And perhaps one Proof of it may be my writing this Eſſay. not intended as a Complaint againſt Providence for my Lot, but as an innocent Amuſement to myſelf and others.

I cannot tell what Effect Deformity may have on the Health but it is natural to imagine, that as the inward Parts of the Body muſt in ſome meaſure comply with the outward Mould, the Form of the

latter

latter being irregular, the firſt cannot be ſo well placed and diſpoſed to perform their Functions and that generally deformed Perſons would not be healthy or long-lived. But this is a Queſtion beſt determined by Facts and in this Caſe the Inſtances are too few, or unobſerved, to draw a general Concluſion from them. And Health is, more than is commonly thought, in a Man's own Power, and the Reward of Temperance, more than the Effect of Conſtitution which makes it ſtill more difficult to paſs a Judgment *Æſop* could not be young when he died and might have lived longer, if he had not been murdered at *Delphos* The Prince of *Orange* ſcarce paſſed the Meridian of Life and the Duke of *Luxemburg* died about the Age of ſixty-ſeven The Lord Treaſurer *Burleigh* (the Honour of whoſe Company I claim on the Authority of * *Osborn*) lived to ſeventy-eight but his Son the Earl of *Saliſbury*, who died about fifteen Years after him, could not reach near that Age. I have heard (but I know not if it is true) that Mr *Pope*'s Father was deformed, and he lived to ſeventy-five: whereas the Son died in middle Age; if he may be ſaid to die, whoſe Works are immortal My Father was not deformed, but active, and my Mother a celebrated Beauty, and I, that am ſo unlike them, have lived to a greater Age and daily ſee my Acquaintance, of a ſtronger Frame, quitting the Stage before me.

But I leave it to better Naturaliſts to determine, whether Deformity, abſtractedly conſidered, is prejudicial to Health, for in its Conſequences, I believe, it is moſt commonly an Advantage Deformed Perſons have a leſs Share of Strength than others, and therefore ſhould naturally be more careful to preſerve

it ;

* See Hiſtorical Memoirs of Queen *Elizabeth*, by *Francis. Osborn*, Eſq.

it · and, as Temperance is the great Preservative of Health, it may incline them to be more temperate. I have reason to think that my own weak Frame and Constitution have prolonged my Life to this present Date But I should impose upon my Reader, and affront Heaven, if I ascribed that to Virtue, which took its Rise from Necessity Being of a consumptive Disposition, I was alarmed, when young, with frequent spitting of Blood this made me abstain from Wine and all strong Liquors; which I have now done for near thirty Years But

(Incidit in Scyllam cupiens vitare Carybdin,)

By this I fell into another Misfortune, and the Stone was the Consequence of my drinking raw Water: but Care and Perseverance, with Abstinence, have so far subdued that Distemper, that at present it is but little interruption to my Ease or Happiness. And weak as I am, I daily see many dying before me, who were designed by Nature for a much longer Life. And I cannot but lament, that the Generality of Mankind so wantonly throw away Health (without which * Life is not Life) when it is so much in their own Power to preserve it If every Virtue in its Consequence is its own Reward, Temperance is eminently so; and every one immediately feels its good Effect And I am persuaded, that many might arrive at *Cornaro's* Age, if they did but follow his Example On thinking upon this Subject, I have adopted many Maxims, which to the World will seem Paradoxes, as certain true Geographical Theorems do to those, who are unacquainted with the Globe I hold as Articles of Faith (but which may be condemned as Heresies in many a General Council assembled about a large Table) That the

smallest

---

* *Non est vivere, sed valere, vita* —Mart. l. 6. Ep 70.

fmallest Liquors are beft That there never was a good Bowl of Punch, nor a good Bottle of Champaign, Burgundy, or Claret That the beft Dinner is one Difh. That an Entertainment grows worfe in proportion as the Number of Difhes increafe. That a Faft is better than a Lord Mayor's Feaft. That no Connoiffeur ever underftood good Eating, That no Minifter of State or Ambaffador ever gave a good Entertainment No King ever fat down to a good Table And that the Peafant fares better than the Prince, &c &c &c Being infpired with fuch Sentiments, what Wonder is it, if I fometimes break out into fuch Ejaculations O Temperance ! Thou Goddefs moft worthy to be adored ! Thou Patronefs of Health! Thou Protector of Beauty! Thou Prolonger of Life ! Thou Infurer of Pleafure! Thou Promoter of Bufinefs! Thou Guardian of the Perfon! Thou Preferver of the Underftanding ! Thou Parent of every intellectual Improvement, and of every moral Virtue !

Another great Prefervative of Health is moderate Exercife; which few deformed Perfons can want Strength to Perform. I never chofe long Journeys, and they have been fatiguing to me, but I never found myfelf worfe for Fatigue And (before I was troubled with the Stone) I have on Occafion rid fifty Miles in a Day, or walked near twenty. And, though now flow in my Motions, I can be on my Feet the greateft Part of the Day, and cannot be faid to laid a fedentary Life As a deformed Perfon is not formed for violent Exercife, he is lefs liable to fuch Diforders as are the natural Confequence of it He will alfo efcape many Accidents, to which Men of athletic Make, and who glory in their Strength, are always expofing themfelves, to make Trial and Proof of it. If he cannot carry an Ox, like *Milo*, he will not, like *Milo*, be handcuffed in the Oak, by attempting to rend it. He will

will not be the Man, that shall ride from *London* to *York* in a Day, or to *Windsor* in an Hour, for a Wager, or that shall be perpetually performing surprizing long Journies in a surprising short Time, for no earthly Business, but the Pleasure of relating them. Conscious of his own Weakness, he will be cautious of running into Places or Occasions of Danger. I deny myself some Entertainments, rather than venture into a Crowd, knowing how unequal I am to a Struggle in it and if a Quarrel should arise, how ill am I qualified for such an Encounter One Blow from a * *Slack*, a *Broughton*, or a *Taylor*, would infallibly consign me over to *Charon* Nature too calls on deformed Persons to be careful not to offer such Affronts, as may call them forth into the Field of false Honour, where they cannot acquit themselves well for want of Strength and Agility and they are securer from such Affronts themselves, since others will consider the little Credit they will gain by compelling them to appear on that Scene On the whole I conclude, that Deformity is a Protection to a Man's Health and Person, which (strange as it may appear) are better defended by Feebleness than Strength

Let me now consider the Influence of bodily Deformity on a Man's Fortune. Among the lower Class, he is cut off from many Professions and Employments He cannot be a Soldier, he is under Standard . he cannot be a Sailor, he wants Activity to climb the Rigging he cannot be a Chairman or Porter, he wants Strength to bear the Burthen. In higher Life, he is ill qualified for a Lawyer, he can scarce be seen over the Bar for a Divine, he may drop from his Hassock out of Sight in his Pulpit. The Improvement of the Mind is his proper Province and his Business only such as depends on Ingenuity If he cannot be a Dancing-master to adjust the Heels, he may be a School-master to instruct

B   the

---

* Three famous Boxers or Bruisers in *London*.

the Head He cannot be a graceful Actor on the Stage, but he may produce a good Play He would appear ill as a Herald in a Procession, but may pass as a Merchant on the Exchange He cannot undergo the Fatigues of the Campaign, but he may advise the Operations of it He is designed by Nature, rather to sleep on *Parnassus*, than to descend on the Plains of *Elis* He cannot be crowned at the *Olympic* Games, but may be the *Pindar* to celebrate them He can acquire no Glory by the Sword, but he may by the Pen and may grow famous by only relating those Exploits, which are beyond his Power to imitate

Lord *Bacon* (that extensive and penetrating Genius, who pointed out every Part of Nature for Examination) in his Essay on Deformity says, ' that, ' in their Superiors, it quencheth Jealousy towards ' them, as Persons, that they think they may at ' pleasure despise and it layeth their Competitors ' and Emulators asleep, as never believing they ' should be in a Possibility of Advancement, till ' they see them in Possession ' But it is much to be doubted, whether this is not more than counterballanced by the Contempt of the World, which it requires no mean Parts to conquer For, if (as I have somewhere read) a good Person is a Letter of Recommendation, Deformity must be an Obstruction in the Way to Favour In this respect therefore deformed Persons set out in the World to a Disadvantage, and they must first surmount the Prejudices of Mankind, before they can be upon a Par with others, and must obtain by a Course of Behaviour that Regard, which is paid to Beauty at first sight. When this Point is once gained, the Tables are turned, and then the Game goes in their Favour for others, sensible of their first Injustice to them, no sooner find them better than they expected, than they believe them better than they are. whereas in the

beautiful

beautiful Perſon, they ſometimes find themſelves im-
poſed upon, and are angry that they have worſhip-
ed only a painted Idol   For (again take Lord *Bacon*'s Words) * ' neither is it almoſt ſeen, that very
' beautiful Perſons are otherwiſe of great Virtue .
' they prove accompliſhed, but not of great Spirit ,
' and ſtudy rather Behaviour than Virtue   Whereas
' † deformed Perſons, if they be of Spirit, will free
' themſelves from Scorn, which muſt be either by
' Virtue or Malice , and therefore let it not be mar-
' velled, if they ſometimes prove excellent Perſons,
' as was *Ageſilaus, Zanger* the Son of *Solomon, Eſop,*
' *Gaſca* Preſident of *Peru* , and *Socrates* may like-
' wiſe go amongſt them, with others ' Nay, he
ſays, ' in a great Wit Deformity is an Advantage to
' Riſing ' And, § in another Part of his Works,
' that they, who by Accident have ſome inevitable
' and indelible Mark on their Perſons or Fortunes,
' as deformed Perſons, Baſtards, &c if they want
' not Virtue, generally prove fortunate '

    Oſborn in his *Hiſtorical Memoirs of Queen Eliza-
beth* informs us , that ' ſhe choſe the goodlieſt Per-
' ſons for her Houſehold Servants , but in her Coun-
' ſellors did not put by Sufficiency, tho' accompa-
' nied by a crooked Perſon , as it chanced in a
' ‖ Father and Son of the *Cecils,* both incomparable
' for Prudence ' It is well known, the Queen would
make the Father *(Burleigh)* ſit in her Preſence , tell-
ing him that ſhe did not uſe him for his Legs, but
Head   But the Son (afterwards Lord Treaſurer and
Earl of *Saliſbury)* was not ſo civilly treated by the
Populace , and is an Inſtance, not only that Envy
purſues a great Man, but that the higheſt Poſt can-

         not

---

* H s Eſſay on Beauty
† His Eſſay on Deformity
§ *De Augmentis Scientiarum,* 1 8 c 2.
‖ I ſuppoſe what *Cambden* ſays of Lord *Burleigh*'s comely and
pleaſing Aſpect relates to his Countenance only

not redeem a deformed one from Contempt , it attends him like his Shadow, and like that too is ever reminding him of his ill Figure , which is often objected for want of real Crimes. For the fame Writer * fays of the fame great Man , ‘ that the Misfortunes accompanying him from his Birth did ‘ not a little add to that Cloud of Detraction, that ‘ fell upon all that he faid or did a Mulct in Nature, like an Optick Spectacle, multiplying much ‘ in the fight of the People the Apparitions of Ill ’ Nor was this Contempt buried with him it trampled on his Afhes, and infulted his Grave , as appears by an Epitaph, which *Ofborn* cites, as void of Wit, as it is full of Scurrility in one Line of which there is an Epithet, not fo elegant, as defcriptive of his ‘ Perfon, *viz.* ‘ Little *Boffive* Robin, that was fo ‘ great ’

Such Contempt in general, joined with the Ridicule of the Vulgar, is another certain Confequence of bodily Deformity For Men naturally defpife what appears lefs beautiful or ufeful and their Pride is gratified, when they fee fuch Foils to their own Perfons It is this Senfe of Superiority, which is teftified by Laughter in the lower fort while their Betters, who know how little any Man whatfoever hath to boaft of, are reftrained by good Senfe and good Breeding from fuch an Infult But it is not eafy to fay why one Species of Deformity fhould be more ridiculous than another, or why the Mob fhould be more merry with a crooked Man, than one that is deaf, lame, fquinting, or purblind Or why fhould they back-bite me (if I may ufe the Expreffion) to my Face, and not laugh at my Face itfelf for being harrowed by the Small-Pox It is a Back in Alto Relievo that bears all the Ridicule , though one would think a prominent Belly a more reafonable Object of it , fince the laft is generally the Effect

of

of Intemporance, and of a Man's own Creation. *Socrates* was ugly, but not contemned ; and * *Philopœmen* of very mean Appearance, and though contemned on that Account, not ridiculed, for † *Montaigne* says, ' Ill Features are but a superficial Ugli-
' ness, and of little Certainty in the Opinion of
' Men . but a Deformity of Limbs is more substan-
' tial, and strikes deeper in ' As it is more uncommon, it is more remarkable and that perhaps is the true Reason, why it is more ridiculed by the Vulgar.

Since this is the Case , I appeal to my Fraternity, whether it is not found Policy to use Stratagem to guard against their Attacks as much as may be , and, since they are deceived by outward Appearances, to call in the Aid of the Taylor, to present them with better Shapes than Nature has bestowed. Against so unfair an Adversary such Fraud is justifiable , tho' I do not approve of it in general. When I was a Child, I was drawn like a Cupid, with a Bow and Arrow in my Hands, and a Quiver on my Shoulder I afterwards thought this an Abuse, which ought to be corrected and when I sat for my Picture some Years ago, I insisted on being drawn as I am, and that the strong Marks of the Small-Pox might appear in my Face , for I did not choose to colour over a Lye. The Painter, said, he never was allowed such Liberty before ; and I advised him, if he hoped to be in Vogue, never to assume it again · for Flatterers succeed best in the World ; and of all Flatterers Painters are the least liable to be detected by those they flatter Nor are the Ladies the only Persons concerned for their Looks.

B 3 *Alex-*

---

* Coming to an Inn, where he was expected, before his Attendants, the Mistress of the House, seeing a plain Person, of very mean Aspect, ordered him to assist in getting Things ready for *Philopœmen* His Attendants finding him so employed, he told them, he was then paying the Tribute of his Ugliness *Plutarch*

† In his Essay on Phisiognomy.

' * *Alexander* chose to have his Picture drawn by
' *Apelles*, and his Statue formed by *Lysippus* And
' the *Spartan Agesilaus* (conscious of his ill Figure)
' would never suffer any Picture or Statue of him to
' be taken He was one of the most considerable
' Persons of his Age both for civil and military
' Virtues, insomuch that he justly acquired the Ap-
' pellation of *Agesilaus* the Great But tho' Nature
' had been uncommonly liberal to him in the nobler
' Endowments of the Mind, she had treated him
' very unfavourably in those of the Body He was
' remarkably low of Stature had one Leg shorter
' than the other, and so very despicable a Counte-
' nance, that he never failed of raising Contempt
' in those, who were unacquainted with his moral
' and intellectual Excellencies It is no wonder
' therefore, that he was unwilling to be delivered
' down to Posterity under the Disadvantages of so
' unpromising a Figure' I have given the † Words
of a late very elegant Translation of *Cicero*'s Letters.
On the whole, I could wish, that Mankind would
be more candid and friendly with us, and, instead
of ridiculing a distorted Person, would rally the Ir-
regularities of the Mind, which are generally as visible as those of the Person, but being more common, they pass with little Notice as well in high as
low Life. § *Mæcenas* would laugh at any Irregula-
rity.

---

* Edicto vetuit, ne quis se præter Apellen
  Pingeret, aut alius Lysippo duceret æra
  Fortis Alexandri vultum simulania —*Hor Ep.* 1 *l* 2
See too Cicero's celebrated Epistle to Lucceius
† From the Translation, and Notes, of the Epistle I have
mentioned
  § Si curtatus inæquali tonsore capillos
    Occurri, rides si forte subucula pexæ
    Trita subest tunicæ, vel si toga dissidet impar,
    Rides quid, mea cum pugnat sententia secum ?
    Quod petiit spernit, repetit quod nuper omisit ?
    Æstuat, et vitæ disconvenit ordine toto ?
    Diruit, ædificat mutat quadrata rotundis ?
    Insanire putas solennia me, neque rides.

rity in *Horace*'s Dreſs, but not any Caprice in his Behaviour, becauſe it was common and faſhionable ſo a Man's Perſon, which is the Dreſs of his Soul, only is ridiculed, while the vicious Qualities of it eſcape ----Let me add, that if ridiculing another's Perſon is in no Caſe to be juſtified, the ill Treatment of it muſt be highly criminal what then muſt we think of *Balbus*, a *Roman* Quæſtor in *Spain*, who wantonly expoſed to wild Beaſts a certain noted Auctioneer at *Seville*, for no other Reaſon, but becauſe he was deformed This is related in a * Letter to *Cicero* by *Aſinius Pollio*, the moſt accompliſhed Gentleman of that Age , who calls *Balbus* a Monſter for this and other Acts of Barbarity I am glad he has preſerved the Memory of this poor Man , whom I here conſecrate to Fame , and place foremoſt in the glorious Liſt of our Martyrs

I will now follow Lord *Bacon* as my Guide, in tracing out ſuch Paſſions and Affections, as moſt naturally reſult from Deformity for he ſays, ' There ' certainly is a Conſent between the Body and the ' Mind, and where Nature erreth in the one, ſhe ' ventureth in the other, and therefore Deformity ' may be beſt conſidered, in this reſpect, as a Cauſe ' which ſeldom fails of the Effect, and not as a Sign, ' which is more deceivable, for as there is an Electi- ' on in Man touching the Frame of his Mind, the ' Stars of natural Inclination are ſometimes eclipſed ' by the Sun of Diſcipline and Virtue '

He begins with ſaying, that ' deformed Perſons ' are commonly even with Nature, for as Nature ' hath done ill by them, ſo do they by Nature, be- ' ing for the moſt part (as the Scripture ſaith) *void* ' *of natural Affection* ' I can neither find out this Paſſage in Scripture, nor the Reaſon of it. nor can

I give

---

* The 7th of the 15th Book in the Tranſlation—the 32d of the 10th in the Original

I give my Affent or Negative to a Propofition, till I am well acquainted with the Terms of it   If by natural Affection is here meant univerfal Benevolence, and Deformity necessarily implies a want of it, a deformed Perfon muft then be a complete Monfter   But however common the Cafe may be, my own Senfations inform me, that it is not univerfally true   If by natural Affection is meant a partial Regard for Individuals , I believe the Remark is judicious, and founded in human Nature   Deformed Perfons are defpifed, ridiculed, and ill-treated by others , are feldom Favourites, and commonly moft neglected by Parents, Guardians, and Relations and therefore, as they are not indebted for much Fondnefs, it is no wonder if they repay but little   It is the Command of Scripture, *Not to fet our Affections on Things below* , which we muft foon part with   and therefore, to be fo fond of others, as not to be able to bear their Abfence, or to furvive them, is neither a religious or moral Duty , but a childifh and womanifh Weaknefs and I muft congratulate deformed Perfons, who by Example are early taught another Leffon   And I will now lay open my own Heart to the Reader, that he may judge, if Lord *Bacon*'s Pofition is verified in me

I hope it proceeds not from a Malignity of Heart; but I never am much affected with the common Accidents of Life, whether they befall myfelf or others. I am little moved when I hear of Death, Lofs, or Misfortune , I think the Cafe is common,

(* *Tritus, et e medio fortunæ ductus acervo :*)

And as it is always likely to happen, I am not furprifed when it does   If I fee a Perfon cry or beat his Breaft on fuch an Occafion, I cannot bear him Company, but am not a *Democritus* to laugh at his Folly   I read of Battles and Fields covered with Slain, of Cities deftroyed by Sword, Famine, Peftilence, and Earthquake , I do not fhed a Tear   I

fuppofe

* Juv. Sat. 13.

suppofe it is, becaufe they are the ufual Storms, to which the human Species are expofed, proceeding from the juft Judgments of God, or the miftaken and falfe Principles of Rulers I read of Perfecutions, Tortures, Murders, Maffacres, my Compaffion for the Sufferers is great, but my Tears are ftopped by Refentment and Indignation againft the Contrivers and Perpetrators of fuch horrid Actions, But there are many Things, that bring Tears into my Eyes, whether I will or no and when I reflect, I am often at a Lofs in fearching out the fecret Source from whence they flow What makes me weep? (for weep I do) when I read of Virtue or Innocence in Diftrefs, of a good Man, helplefs and forfaken, unmoved by the greateft Infults and Cruelties, or courageoufly fupporting himfelf againft Oppreffion in the Article of Death I fuppofe it is, to fee Vice triumphant, and Virtue fo ill rewarded in this Life. May I judge by myfelf, I fhould imagine, that few fincere *Chriftians* could read the Sufferings of their *Saviour*, or *Englifhmen* thofe of a *Cranmer*, *Ridley*, or *Latimer*, without Tears ; the firft dying to eftablifh his Religion, the laft to refcue it from Corruption When I read of * *Regulus* returning to Torment, and † *John* of *France* to Imprifonment, againft the Perfuafion of Friends, to keep Faith with their Enemies ; I weep to think, there is fcarce an-

other

* Donec labantes confilio patres
Firmaret auctor nunquam alias dato,
Interque mœrentes amicos
Egregius properaret exul.
Atqui fciebat quæ fibi barbarus
Tortor pararet ———— tamen
Dimovit obftantes propinquos,
Et populum reditus morantem

Hor Od 5 1 3

† En vain fes Miniftres & les plus confiderables Seigneurs du Royaume firent tous leurs efforts, pour le faire changer de refolution Il repondoit à tout ce qu'on lui difoit là deffus, que quand la bonne foy feroit bannie du refte du monde, il falloit qu'on la trouvat toujours dans la bouche des Rois. Hiftoire de *France*, par le *P G Daniel*

other Inftance of fuch exalted Virtue. Thofe, who often hear me read, know, that my Voice changes, and my Eyes are full, when I meet with a generous and heroic Saying, Action, or Character, efpecially of Perfons, whofe Example or Command may influence Mankind. I weep when I hear a * *Titus* fay, That he had loft the Day in which he did no Good. When † *Adrian* tells his Enemy, That he had efcaped by his being Emperor, or § *Lewis* XII. That he is not to revenge the Affronts of the Duke of *Orleans*. Thefe are the firft Inftances that happen to occur to me. I might collect many, too many to infert in this Effay, yet all are but few, compared to Inftances of Cruelty and Revenge. perhaps I am concerned, that they are fo rare. perhaps too I inwardly grieve, that I am not in a Situation to do the like. I am entertained, but not moved, when I read *Voltaire*'s Hiftory of *Charles* XII. but I melt into Tears on reading *Hanway*'s Character of his Antagonift *Peter* the Great. The firft is the Story of a Madman, the other of a Father, Friend, and Benefactor of his People, whofe Character (as the Author obferves in the Conclufion of it) will command the Admiration of all fucceeding Generations· and I fuppofe I lament, that God is pleafed to advance to Royalty fo few fuch Inftruments of Good to Mankind. *Henry* IV of *France* had every Quality to make a Prince amiable, Courage, Humanity, Clemency, Generofity, Affability, Politenefs· his Behaviour on every Occafion is charming. and I cannot read the Account of him, given us by his Prime Minifter (*Sully*,) without Emotion. I do not wonder, if what is reported is true, that ‖ at leaft

fifty

---

* Recordatus quondam fuper cœnam, quod nihil cuiquam to o die præftitiffet, memorabilem illam meritoque laudatam vocem cœidit AMICI DIEM PERDIDI Suetonius

† Echard's Roman Hiftory

§ Mezerai, & Daniel

‖ Moreri's Dictionary.—Turkifh Spy, Vol. I B. 2. Let. 20

fifty Perfons have written his Hiftory , and that he has been celebrated in Poems, and Panegyricks, by above five hundred   there are few fuch Subjects to be met with , and few Princes, who have fo juftly deferved the Title of Great   His Grandfon had the fame Title beftowed on him   but how little did he deferve it! He has been celebrated by as many Hiftoriographers and Poets , but they are moftly fuch as he hired for that Purpofe   and none of them, even *Voltaire* himfelf, will be able to pafs him for a great Man on unprejudiced Pofterity   Compare him with his Grandfather, you will find him the Reverfe. *Henry* was bred to Toil and Hardfhips , *Lewis* in Luxury and Effeminacy   *Henry* pleafant, eafy, and affable , *Lewis* formal, haughty, and referved. *Henry* brave, and expofing himfelf to all Dangers , *Lewis* cautious, and always in a fecure Poft   The one gaining Victories by himfelf, and his own perfonal Valour , the other by his Generals, and Superiority of Numbers   The one pleafed with performing great Actions, the other with being flattered for thofe which he never performed   The firft ambitious of true, and the laft of falfe Glory   *Henry* ftabbed by Jefuits , *Lewis* governed by them   The one forgiving Rebels and Affaffins , the other encouraging both   *Henry* perfecuted , *Lewis* a Perfecutor   The firft granting Liberty of Confcience , the laft taking it away   *Herry* promoting the Silk Manufacture in *France* , *Lewis* in *England*   One treating his Subjects as his Children , the other as his Slaves   *Henry* bravely afferting his own Rights , *Lewis* bafely encroaching on thofe of his Neighbours   *Henry* extricating his Country from Mifery, and laying the Foundation of her Grandeur , *Lewis* fquandering her Blood and Treafure, and reducing her from Grandeur to the Brink of Deftruction. *Henry* forming Schemes for the perpetual Peace of *Europe* ;

Lewis

Lewis perpetually to difturb it   How little is *Lewis*
compared to *Henry* the Great !

But to return to my Subject. ————I am uneafy
when I fee a Dog, a Horfe, or any other Animal ill
treated , for I confider them as endued with quick
Senfe, and no contemptible Share of Reafon , and
that God gave Man Dominion over them, not to
play the Tyrant, but to be a good Prince and promote the Happinefs of his Subjects   But I am much
more uneafy at any Cruelty to my own Species , and
heartily wifh *Procruftes* difciplined in his own Bed,
and *Phalaris* in his Bull.   A Man bruifed all over in
a Boxing Match, or cut to Pieces in fighting a Prize,
is a fhocking Spectacle , and I think I could with
lefs Horror fee a thoufand fall in Battle, than human
Nature thus depreciated and difgraced   Violence,
when exerted in Wantonnefs or Paffion, is Brutality :
and can be termed Bravery, only when it is fanctified
by Juftice and Neceffity.   A mangled Carcafs is not
a pleafing Sight.   Why therefore do Men pay for
it ? and the great Vulgar encourage thefe Diforders
among the Small ? It is not Choice, but Affectation.
As many, who neither love nor underftand Mufick,
go to an Opera to gain the Reputation of Connoi-
feurs , many go to *Broughton*'s Theatre, to avoid the
Imputation of being Cowards   but when they are at
fo much Pains to avoid the Imputation, it raifes a
Sufpicion that they are fo

I have been in a Situation to fee not a little of the
Pomp and Vanity, as well as of the Neceffity and
Mifery of Mankind   but the laft only affect me :
and if, as a Magiftrate, I am ever guilty of Parti-
ality, it is in favour of the Poor   When I am at
Church among my poor, but honeft, Neighbours
in the Country , and fee them ferious in performing
the Ceremonies prefcribed , Tears fometimes fteal
down my Cheek, on reflecting that they are doing
and hearing many Things they do not underftand ;

while

while thofe who underſtand them better neglect
them   that they who labour and live hard, are more
thankful to Heaven, than thofe who fare luxuriouſly
on the Fruits of their Labour· and are keeping and
repeating the fourth Commandment at the very In-
ſtant the others are breaking it

Thefe are ſome of the Senfations I feel ; which I
have freely and fairly diſcloſed, that the Reader
may judge, how far I am an Inſtance of a deformed Perſon wanting natural Affection   And I am
a good Subject of Speculation , for all in me is Nature   for to own the Truth, I have taken but little
Pains (tho' much I ought to have taken) to correct
my natural Defects

Lord *Bacon*'s next Poſition is, ' That deformed
' Perſons are extremely bold. Firſt in their own
' Defence, as being expoſed to Scorn ; but in Pro-
' ceſs of Time by a general Habit '——This probably is ſo among the inferior Sort, who are in the
Way of continual Inſults   for a Return of Abuſe is
a natural Weapon of Self-defence , and in ſome
meaſure juſtified by the Law of Retaliation   to up-
braid a Man with a perſonal Defect, which he cannot help, is alſo an immoral Act , and he who does
it has reaſon to expect no better Quarter, than to
hear of Faults, which it was in his own Power not
to commit.   But I find this Obſervation far from
being verified in myſelf   an unbecoming Baſhful-
neſs has been the Conſequence of my ill Figure,
and of the worſe Management of me in my Childhood   I am always uneaſy, when any one looks
ſtedfaſtly on ſo bad a Picture , and cannot look
with a proper Confidence in the Face of another.
I have ever reproached myſelf with this Weakneſs,
but am not able to correct it.   And it may be a
Diſadvantage to a Man in the Opinion of thoſe he
converſes with , for though true Modeſty is amiable,
the falſe is liable to Miſconſtruction , and when a

Man

Man is out of Countenance for no Reason, it may be imagined, that he has some bad Reason for being so. In point of Assurance, I am indeed a perfect Riddle to myself: for I, who feel a Reluctance in crossing a Drawing-room, or in opening my Mouth in private Company before Persons with whom I am not well acquainted, find little in delivering my Sentiments in Public, and exposing my Discourse, often as trifling as my Person, to the Ears of a Thousand. From what Cause this proceeds I know not: it may be, partly from Hopes of wiping off any ill Impressions from my Person by my Discourse, partly from a Sense of doing my Duty, and partly from a Security in publick Assemblies from any gross personal Reflections.

Lord *Bacon* compares the Case of deformed Persons to that of Eunuchs, ' in whom Kings were ' wont to put great Trust as good Spials and Whis- ' perers, for they, that are envious towards all, are ' more obnoxious and officious towards one.' But with Submission to so good a Judge of human Nature, I own, I can discover no uncommon Qualifications in them for Spies, and very few Motives to Envy peculiar to themselves. Spies submit to that base and ungenerous Office, either for the Sake of Interest or Power: if for Interest, it is to gratify their Covetousness, if for Power, their Ambition or Revenge: which Passions are not confined to the Eunuch or Deformed, but indiscriminately seize all Classes of Men. Envy too may prompt a Man to mean Actions, in order to bring down the Person envied to his own Level, but, if it is on account of Superiority of Fortune, it will operate alike on Men of all Shapes. Eunuchs have but one peculiar Motive to Envy: but that (as Lord *Bacon* expresses it) makes them envious towards all, because it is for a Pleasure, which all but themselves may enjoy. Deformed Persons are deprived only

of

of Beauty and Strength, and therefore thofe alone
are to be deemed the extraordinary Motives to their
Envy , for they can no more be beautiful or ftrong,
than Eunuchs be fuccefsful Lovers   As to myfelf ,
whatever Sparks of Envy might be in my Conftitu-
tion, they are now entirely extinguifhed   for by
frequent and ferious Reflection I have long been con-
vinced of the fmall Value of moft Things which
Men value the moft.

There is another Paffion to which deformed Perfons feem to be more expofed, than to Envy , which
is Jealoufy   for being confcious, that they are lefs
amiable than others, they may naturally fufpect, that
they are lefs beloved   I have the Happinefs to
fpeak this from Conjecture, and not from Experience   for it was my Lot many Years ago to marry
a young Lady, very pioufly educated, and of a very
diftinguifhed Family, and whofe Virtues are an Honour to her Family, and her Sex   fo that I had
never any Trial of my Temper , and can only guefs
at it by Emotions I have felt in my younger Days ;
when Ladies have been more liberal of their Smiles
to thofe, whom I thought in every refpect, but Perfon, my Inferiors

The moft ufeful Inference from all this to a deformed Perfon is, to be upon his Guard againft
thofe Frailties, to which he is more particularly expofed, and to be careful, that the outward Frame
do not diftort the Soul * *Orandum eft*, let us pray,
fays *Juvenal*, *ut fit mens fana in corpore fano*, for a
found Mind in a healthy Body , and every deformed
Perfon fhould add this Petition, *ut fit mens recta in
corpore curvo*, for an upright Mind in a crooked one
And let him frequently apply to himfel, this Article of Self-examination, † *Lenior & melior fis acce-
dente fenectâ ?* As Age approaches, do your Temper
and

and Morals improve? It is a Duty peculiarly incumbent for if Beauty adds Grace to Virtue itself, Vice muft be doubly hideous in Deformity.

Ridicule and Contempt are a certain Confequence of Deformity and therefore what a Perfon cannot avoid, he fhould learn not to regard He fhould bear it like a Man, forgive it as a Chriftian, and confider it as a Philofopher. And his Triumph will be complete, if he can exceed others in Pleafantry on himfelf Wit will give over when it fees itfelf out-done, and fo will Malice, when it finds it has no Effect and if a Man's Behaviour afford no Caufe of Contempt, it will fall upon thofe, who contemn him without Caufe It fometimes happens, that Perfons, with whom I have a flight Acquaintance, will take notice of me on fome Days, and overlook me on others, well knowing, that they ought to treat one of my Shape, with the precife degree of Ceremony, which fuits their prefent Humour. I will not fay, this is a Pleafure, but I can truly fay, it is no Mortification. It excites in me no Refentment, but only Speculation and not able to find out a very good Reafon for their Behaviour, I endeavour to find out as good a one as I can I confider with myfelf, what it is, which makes them at that Juncture of fuch particular Importance to themfelves and afk myfelf many Queftions of this Sort Is his Father dead? Has he writ a Play? Has he dined with my Lord Mayor? Has he made a Speech? Has he been prefented at Court? Has he been fpoke to at a Levee? Has he a new Equipage or Title? Has he had a good Run? Has he got a Place? Is he gone to marry a Fortune? Has he been congratulated on the Performance of his *French* Cook, or his *French* Taylor? Is he reckoned a Man of Tafte? Is he admitted of *White*'s, or of the Royal Society?——Such are the Topicks of my Speculations. and though I am a

Perfon

Person of no great Penetration, I sometimes hit on the right Cause.

Fine Cloaths attract the Eyes of the Vulgar and therefore a deformed Person should not assume those borrowed Feathers, which will render him doubly ridiculous He could scarce expose himself more by dancing at Court, than by appearing the finest there on a Birth-day Ever since I arrived at Years of Discretion, I have worn a plain Dress, which, for near thirty Years, has been of the same grave Colour, and which I find not the least Inclination to alter. It would be monstrous in me to bestow any Ornament on a Person, which is incapable of it and should I appear in Lace or Embroidery, my Friends might assign it as no unreasonable Pretence for a Commission of Lunacy against me —— I can scarce forbear digressing on this Subject, when I reflect, what Numbers, who should know better, set a Value upon these Trifles, which are fit Amusements only for Children If they are pleased with the Finery only, they are no better than Children. If it is to gain Respect, such Respect must come from the Vulgar, and not from Men of Sense Is it to shew their Quality? it does not, for even Apprentices are fine Is it to be an Evidence of their Riches? it is not, for the most necessitous are finest, as Taylors know to their Cost. Do their Figure or Reputation depend on their Dress? then they are entirely in the Hands of the Taylor he is the Engineer to guard and defend them, the God to save or destroy Do they dress to please the Ladies? that is the most reasonable End yet very few of them but are wiser than to be taken with the Coat instead of the Man and what can be taking in a Man who invades their Province, and appears by his Actions to be one of them?—If it is a Lady that is fond of Finery, I ask her why? If she is a Beauty, she wants no Ornament if plain, she can-

C

not

not be transformed. Her dreſs indeed may enliven her Poet's Fancy, and ſave him a Journey to the Sun and Stars for his Similes and Alluſions. If the Lady had not put on her Finery, we might have loſt this polite and ingenious Stanza,

> *The adorning thee with ſo much Art*
> *Is but a barbarous Skill*
> *'Tis like the poiſoning of a Dart,*
> *Too apt before to kill.*

Every Mother (like her in * *Juvenal*) hath pray-ed in the Temple of *Venus* for the moſt exquiſite Beauty in her Children. But ſince the Goddeſs hath been thus deaf and unkind, I cannot adviſe any one of my Sex to be her profeſt Votary. for ſhe will be as little propitious to his Wiſhes, as ſhe was to his Mother's Prayer A *Helen* will run away with a *Paris·* but where is the Nymph, that will liſten to ſuch a *Corydon?* In vain will he ſummon the Muſes to his Aid, unaſſiſted as he is by the Graces His † *Sachariſſa, Myra, Cloe,* or *Belinda,* may per-haps tickle her Ear, but will never touch her Heart

> § *Not Words alone pleaſe her.*

Or if (as ‖ *Waller* expreſſes it) her high Pride ſhould deſcend to mark his Follies, it is the greateſt Ho-nour he can expect· unleſs in a merry Mood ſhe ſhould take into her Head to treat him like ** *Fal-ſtaff* or Squire *Slender.* He will be the choiceſt of
Cupid's

---

* Formam optat modico pueris, majore puellis
  Murmure cùm Veneris ſanum videt anxia mater,
  Uſque ad delicias votorum ——— *Sat* 10
† *Sachariſſa* belongs to *Waller, Myra* to *Landſdown, Cloe* to *Prior,* and *Belinda* to *Pope*
§ Milton Par Loſt b 8.
‖ In his Poem on Love.
** Merry Wives of Windſor

Cupid's April Fools; and I will not fay an egregious Afs, but Camel, to bear his Burthens But let this be fome Confolation to him, that while he is not fuffered to regale on the Sweets of the Hive, he is fecured from its Sting.

But, not to make ugly Perfons out of Love with themfelves, I will now exhibit fome Advantages arifing from Deformity.

Inftead of repining, a deformed Perfon ought to be thankful to Providence for giving him fuch a Guard to his Virtue and Repofe Thoufands are daily ruined by a handfome Perfon for Beauty is a Flower that every one wants to gather in its Bloom, and fpares no Pains or Stratagem to reach it. All the Poetical Stories concerning it have their Moral A *Helen* occafions War and Confufion. The *Hyacinths* and *Ganimedes* are feized on for Catamites the *Endymions* and *Adonifes* for Gallants *Narciffus* can admire no body but himfelf, and grows old, before he is cured of that Paffion Who is a Stranger to the Story of *Lucretia*, killing herfelf for her violated Chaftity? or of *Virginia*, killed by her Father to preferve it? in thofe Circumftances, fays * *Juvenal*, fhe might wifh to change Perfons with *Rutila*, the only Lady I know among the Ancients celebrated for a Hump-Back. The † handfomeft Men are chofen for Eunuchs and Gallants· and when they are catched in exercifing the laft Function, both § *Horace*

C 2   and

---

* Sed vetat optari faciem Lucretia, qualem
  Ipfa habuit Cuperet Rutilæ Virginia gibbum
  Accipere, atque fuam Rutilæ dare ——Sat. 10
       † ——Nullus ephebum
  Deformem fæva caftravit in arce tyrannus
  Nec pretextatum rapuit Nero loripedem, nec
  Strumofum, atque utero pariter gibboque tumentem
                                      ibid

§ Hic fe præcipitem tecto dedit ille flagellis
  Ad mortem cæfus fugiens hic decidit acrem
  Prædonum in turbam dedit hic pro corpore nummos
                                      Hunc

and *Juvenal* inform you of the Penalties and Indignities they undergo   * *Silius* was converted by the insatiable *Messalina* into a Husband   and *Sporus* by the Monster † *Nero* into a Wife   The last mentioned Poet shews, that praying for Beauty is praying for a Curse   and § *Persius* refuses to join in such a Prayer   and have not I reason to thank my Stars, that have placed me more out of Danger than even Virtue could , for that could not guard a ‖ *Joseph*, an ** *Hippolytus*, a *Bellerophon*, and others, against the Revenge of slighted Love.

Another great Advantage of Deformity is, that it tends to the improvement of the Mind   A Man, that cannot shine in his Person, will have recourse to his Understanding, and attempt to adorn that Part of him, which alone is capable of Ornament

when

Hunc perminxerunt calones   quinet am illud
Accidit, ut cuidam testes caudamque salacem
Demeteret ferrum ——————— Hor Sat 2 1 1
———Quosdam mæchos & mugilis intrat   Juv ibid
* ———Optimus hic & formosissimus idem
Gentis Patriciæ rapitur miser extinguendus
Messalinæ oculis ———— Juv Sat 10
† Suetonius
§ Hunc optent generum Rex & Regina   puellæ
Hunc rapiant quicquid calcaverit hic, rosa fiat
Ast ego nutrici non mando vota , negato
Jupiter hæc illi ———— Pers Sat 2
‖   Gen c 39
**   — Quid profuit olim
Hippolito grave propositum ? Quid Bellerophonti ?
Erubuit nempe hæc, seu fastidita repulsâ
Nec Sthenobœa minus quam Cressa excanduit, & se
Concussere ambæ —— Juv Sat 10
Ut Prætum mulier perfida credulum
Falsis impulerit criminibus, nimis
Casto Bellerophonti
Maturare necem, refert
Narrat penè datum Pelea Tartaro,
Magnessam Hippolyten dum fugit abstinens
Hor Od 7 1 3

when his Ambition prompts him to begin with *Cowley*, to afk himfelf this Queftion,

> *What fhall I do to be for ever known*
> *And make the Age to come my own?*

On looking about him, he will find many Avènues to the Temple of Fame barred againft him but fome are ftill open through that of Virtue and thofe, if he has a right Ambition, he will moft probably attempt to pafs The more a Man is unactive in his Perfon, the more his Mind will be at work and the Time which others fpend in Action, he will pafs in Study and Contemplation by thefe he may acquire Wifdom, and by Wifdom Fame. The Name of *Socrates* is as much founded, as thofe of *Alexander* and *Cæfar*, and is recorded in much fairer Characters He gained Renown by Wifdom and Goodnefs, they by Tyranny and Oppreffion he by inftructing, they by deftroying Mankind · and happy it is that their evil Deeds were confined to their Lives, while he continues to inftruct us to this this Day A deformed Perfon will naturally confider, where his Strength and his Foible lie ; and as he is well acquainted with the laft, he will eafily find out the firft, and muft know, that (if it is any where) it is not, like *Sampfon's*, in the Hair , but muft be in the lining of the Head He will fay to himfelf, I am weak in Perfon , unable to ferve my Country in the Field , I can acquire no military Glory . but I may, like *Socrates*, acquire Reputation by Wifdom and Probity let me therefore be wife and honeft My Figure is very bad, and I fhould appear but ill as an Orator, either in the Pulpit or at the Bar let me therefore pafs my Time in my Study, either in reading what may improve myfelf, or in writing what may entertain or inftruct others. I have not the Strength of *Hercules*, nor

can

can I rid the World of so many Monsters · but perhaps I may get rid of some myself If I cannot
draw out *Cacus* from his Den, I may pluck the Vil-
lain from my own Breast I cannot cleanse the
Stables of *Augeas*, but I may cleanse my own
Heart from Filth and Impurity I may demolish
the *Hydra* of Vices within me, and should be careful too, * that while I lop off one, I do not suffer
more to grow up in its stead Let me be serviceable
in any way that I can : and if I am so, it may in
some measure be owing to my Deformity Which at
least should be a Restraint on my Conduct, lest my
Conduct make me more deformed.

Few Persons have a House entirely to their Mind ;
or the Apartment in it disposed as they could wish.
And there is no deformed Person, who does not
wish, that his Soul had a better Habitation, which
is sometimes not lodged according to its Quality.
Lord *Clarendon* says of Sir *Charles Cavendish* (Brother to the Marquess of *Newcastle*) that he was a Man
of the noblest and largest Mind, though of the least
and most inconvenient Body, that lived And
every body knows, that the late Prince of *Orange*
had many amiable Qualities. Therefore in Justice
to such Persons I must suppose, that they did not
repine, that their Tenements were not in a more regular Style of Architecture And let every deformed Person comfort himself with reflecting, that tho'
his Soul hath not the most convenient and beautiful Apartment, yet that it is habitable that the Ac-
commodation will serve in an Inn upon the Road
that he is but Tenant for Life, or (more properly)
at Will · and that, while he remains in it, he is in
a State to be envied by the Deaf, the Dumb, the
Lame, and the Blind

When

* Quid te exempta juvat spinis de pluribus una ?
Hor Ep 2 | 2

When I die, I care not what becomes of the contemptible Carcaſs, which is the Subject of this Eſſay I wonder at the Weakneſs of ſome of the old Patriarchs, that provided burying Places, that their Bones might be gathered to their Fathers. Doth one Clod of Earth delight in the Neighbourhood of another? or is there any Converſation in the Grave? It muſt have been a Joke in Sir *Samuel Garth*, when he ordered himſelf and Lady to be buried at *Harrow on the Hill* one of his Strength of Mind could have no Superſtition of that Sort. It is of no Conſequence where the Body rots · whether it rots immediately, or be preſerved a few Years or whether it be devoured by Birds or Beaſts, or placed in a Sumptuous Tomb If a Man doth not provide himſelf a Monument by his Actions, and embalm his Memory in Virtue, the lying Marble will decay, and then his Memorial (even in that little Corner) will periſh,

* *Quandoquidem data ſunt ipſis quoque fata ſepulchris*

The *Pharaohs* are ſtolen from their Pyramids ; and their Mummies diſperſed thro' the World only as idle Curioſities. And tho' the Pyramids are more durable than common Sepulchres, yet their Hiſtory is already unknown, and they muſt in the End undergo the ſame Fate. † Mr *Addiſon* admires the Humanity of *Cyrus* (or rather *Xenophon*) in ordering his Body to be buried in the Earth, that it might be uſeful in manuring it My Fleſh will afford but little Manure · but in another Reſpect my Carcaſs may be of eminent Service to Mankind · and therefore if I ſhould die inteſtate, or not mention it in my Will, let the World take this as my dying Requeſt.

* Juv Sat 10
† Spectator, Nº 169

queſt   As I have for ſome Years been afflicted with
the * Stone, and owe the Preſervation and Eaſe of
Life ſince to the continued taking of great Quanti-
ties of Soap, I deſire my Body may be opened and
examined by eminent Surgeons, that Mankind may
be informed of its Effect.   And if a Stone ſhould
be found in my Bladder (as I imagine there will) I
deſire it may be preſerved among Sir *Hans Sloane*'s
Collection ——Until that Time comes, I hope to
employ the little Remainder of Life in Purſuits not
unbecoming a rational Creature

My CASE.

FOR many Years red Sand conſtantly came from
me without Pain or Inconvenience.   About
nine Years ago I began to be uneaſy   and before
twelve Months had paſſed, was ſo much out of Order, that I could no longer ride, the Motion of a
Coach grew inſupportable, and that of a Chair, or
Walking, was generally attended with bloody Water.

The Regimen.

I took Mrs *Stephens*'s Medicine in the ſolid Form,
three Ounces a Day, for about five Years, when I
changed it for the ſame Quantity of Caſtile Soap,
which about a Year ſince I reduced to two Ounces,
and lately to one Ounce, with about a Pint of Lime-
Water mixt with Milk   being willing to regain my
Liberty, as far as is conſiſtent with Eaſe and Safety
This Regimen I have inceſſantly purſued, except
some

* I will here give a more particular Account of myſelf with
regard to that Diſtemper, which I hope will be of mo e imme-
diate Service

fome few Days that I have purpofely omitted it, to obferve the Confequences of fuch Omiffion.

The Effects.

Whilft I purfue this Regimen, I never difcharge red Sand, whenever I omit it for a few Days, I conftantly do By a fteady Perfeverance in it, my particular Complaint has been gradually diminifhed; and my Health in general improved. I believe I could now ride, tho' I have not tried I feldom feel any Uneafinefs in a Coach, and when I do, it is inconfiderable, tho' fometimes (but very rarely) it is attended with bloody Water And the Motion of a Chair or Walking do not affect me In fhort, I have exchanged Pain for Eafe, and Mifery for Comfort and had it not been for this Medicine, I fhould not have been now alive to have told my Story

My Conclufions are thefe,

1. Mrs *Stephens*'s Medicine or Caftile Soap are fafe Remedies and three Ounces may be taken every Day for Years together (and probably during Life) without any ill Confequence

2 That Health in general will improve by their Ufe for by their cleanfing Quality, I imagine, they better prepare the Stomach for Digeftion, and the Inteftines for Chylification.

3. They are Preventives of the Stone, either by hindering the Generation or Formation of thofe Particles of which it is compofed, or by facilitating the difcharge of them before Concretion And I am perfuaded, that by taking them, Perfons, who have not that Diftemper, will be fecured from it, and thofe, who have it, from growing worfe And if, on leffening my Quantity I again find the Ap-

D

pearance of red Sand, I will increase it again to a Quantity sufficient to prevent it

4 They are Lithentriptics Of this I have often had ocular Proof and the discharged Fragments are softened , and their Parts more easily separated

5 They are Lenitives where the Stone is not entirely discharged so that when a compleat Cure is not obtained, Ease may , as I have happily experienced But from what Cause this proceeds, let Physicians enquire and determine

I believe, Men scarce differ so much in the Temper of their Bodies, as of their Minds and tho' many Cases may be very unlike my own, I am persuaded, that a regular Use of this Medicine would for the most part be as beneficial to others as to myself Persons, with whom it disagrees, in other respects, are excluded from this Benefit as the Intemperate are from the Benefit of this or any other Medicine

I have for a long Course of Years abstained from all strong Liquors, but drink every thing that is small I can eat any thing, but not much , and like the most common Diet best I prefer most things to Flesh , and of Flesh the whitest I never altered my common Diet on Account of this Medicine , or the Times of my Meals, which have been very irregular I have always taken an Ounce at a time , sometimes before, sometimes at, and sometimes after Meals and I have often made a Meal of the Medicine itself, only with a Glass of small Liquor (of any sort) and a little Bread, which I have always taken with it I generally took the three Ounces at proper Intervals , and sometimes at very short ones This Medicine has always agreed with me , and I never once felt it on my Stomach, or any other Inconvenience from it And I think it my Duty to omit no Opportunity of publishing its Virtues to the World.

POST.

POSTSCRIPT.

SINCE I finished this Essay, I am in Doubt whether I ought not to change the Title For I have heard of a very ingenious Performance, called *The Analysis of Beauty*, which proves incontestibly, that it consists in Curve Lines · I congratulate my Fraternity , and hope for the future the Ladies will esteem them *Des Beaux Garçons.*

F I N I S.

	l.	s.	d.
THE Works of Virgil, in Latin and Engliſh. By the Rev Mr Pitt, and the Rev. Mr Wharton In 4 neat Pocket Volumes.	0	13	0
The Rambler, 6 Vols 13s or bound in three	0	11	4
Letters from ſeveral Parts of Europe, and the Eaſt In 2 Volumes	0	6	6
The Letters of Marcus Tullius Cicero to ſeveral of his Friends By William Melmoth, Eſq In 3 neat Pocket Volumes	0	9	9
The Preſent State of Europe	0	5	5
The Spirit of Laws Tranſlated from the French of the celebrated M De Seondat, Baron De Monteſquieu, in 2 Vols 8vo.	0	10	10
Peter Wilkins, 2 Vols 12mo.	4	10	
The Hiſtory of Pompey the Little, or, the Life and Adventures of a Lap Dog		2	2
Chambers's Dictionary, 2 Vols Folio.	4	11	0
Voltaire's Letters concerning the Engliſh Nation, Twelves		2	2
Thoughts on Religion, and other various Subjects, by M Paſcal, Octavo.		4	4
The Pantheon		2	6
The Winter-Evening Tales, containing Seventeen delightful Novels		2	2
Meſſieurs Port-Royais Greek Grammar, recommend-ed by all the Univerſities in Europe		6	6
The Compleat Family Piece, with Directions for Hunting, Hawking, Fiſhing, Fowling, Conſerves, Confectionary, Cookery, Physick and Surgery		3	3
Diſſertation on Parties		2	8
Political Tracts		2	8
Oldcaſtle's Remarks on the Hiſtory of England		2	8
Letters on the Spirit of Patriotiſm		2	2
N. B The four Books abovementioned are writ-ten by the Lord Viſcount Bolingbroke			
Fitz Oſborne's Letters		2	2
Familiar Letters		2	2
SIMPSON's Algebra.	0	6	6
Gordon's Geographical Grammar	0	5	0
Mead on the Small Pox	0	1	1
The Perſeis, or, Secret Memoirs for a Hiſtory of Perſia,	0	2	0

Lightning Source UK Ltd.
Milton Keynes UK
UKHW030928200721
387465UK00010B/1848